The Winning and Healing Mindset

Chinyerem Cynthia Nwachukwu

The Winning and Healing Mindset
How to Maintain Optimal Health and Recover from Sickness. How Health Workers Can Help.

Published by Spines
ISBN: 979-8-89383-655-4

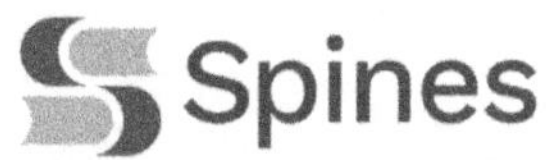

The Winning and Healing Mindset

How to Maintain Optimal Health and Recover from Sickness

How Health Workers Can Help

BY

Chinyerem Cynthia Nwachukwu

Contents

“A very interesting book. It looks small but it's fully loaded. I saw everything I have believed in life now in print. I am greatly optimistic and I am really excited to read about the various studies which you extensively quoted. The book is packed and the size makes one attack it head-on. I read it twice in two days. I recommend it for everyone.”

Emeritus Prof. Frank C. Akpuaka

Professor of Plastic/Reconstructive surgery

and Professor of Anatomy.

"The Winning and Healing Mindset" is solid, clearly written, providing a sensible introduction to the basis of natural health management. The greatest challenge of western medicine is to educate and motivate patients to adopt a healthier lifestyle. This book is doing exactly that,..... with clarity, charm, and thoroughness. I strongly recommend it for everyone.

Prof. Patrick U. Nze

Professor of Anaesthesia

This book is dedicated to all patients whose lifestyles gave an insight into this topic.

Acknowledgments

I appreciate my husband, Dr Amaechi Nwachukwu, children, mum, and siblings for their support, contributions and proof-reading of the manuscript.

I appreciate my teachers at all levels for their labour of love.

I acknowledge the authors whose books gave me a mental shift and enabled me to view life from a broader horizon.

Foreword

Disciplinary public health and community medicine is the specialization in the medical profession that brings medicine and all health practices to meet with every necessary aspects of every profession and job description that exist. Prominent among these are all the essential aspects of the nursing profession; and beyond it, of pharmacy, law, education, engineering, industry, psychology, all the social sciences, etc. In the past as the specialty was developing, through the non-fully post-graduate practices of public health (1374), through preventive and social medicine (1930s) to the full discipline and specialization, less than 50 years ago in 1972, its professionals in their work and writings had concentrated on the strict academic, intellectual and professional needs of their colleagues, clients and communities as structurally existing.

It is therefore quite a delight that younger specialists are now doing their best to fill the entire needs, the services, and the personal and community education that are or can be its privilege and responsibility to provide to the community at large - professionals and the lay public at large. So, it was such a delight for me to learn that Dr. Chinyerem Nwachukwu has decided to toe this very delightful line in her work. It was therefore very satisfying for me to read this her booklet in this regard, for the assistance of one and all in positive psychology and healthy living. I read-studied the booklet in one rapid sweep as it was such a delight to read - content, font size, etc.

I recommend the literature to colleagues in the medical and health professions as an example of the wider health attitude and practice that we should be adopting, and early also in our professional lives; in contrast with the over-clinicalized attitudes, especially where these may obviously be unnecessary. I obviously doubly recommend it to the lay public who clearly are the primary object of the book. I look forward to see both Chinyerem and others, especially younger, colleagues producing more literature of this genre and in greater scope and depth in the immediate years ahead.

Dr. Michael C Asuzu

Professor of Disciplinary Public Health and Community Medicine (retired).

President, Society for Public Health Professionals of Nigeria (SPHPN).

President, Africa Federation of (the National) Public Health Associations (AFPHA).

February, 2024.

Preface

I read a story about a case of diarrhoea which was suspected to be due to food poisoning. The affected individual ate food that he purchased from one of the food stands in a stadium during a game. An announcement was made requesting that people who bought food from the said food stand should not eat it because of the incident. Within minutes, several cases of diarrhoea were reported. Food samples from the food stand were tested and found to be safe. The index case confirmed that he had eaten elsewhere before arriving at the stadium. Then, another announcement was made to counter the first. As expected, many of the cases got better. So, what happened? What we hear affects our bodies and can make us sick or well.

The mind-body connection is a well-established concept, and cultivating positivity in our thoughts and attitudes can have profound effects on our physical health. Controlling what we think about is possible and can be mastered with practice. The benefits are enormous and sometimes mind-blowing.

Positive thinking and a positive mental attitude have emerged as powerful tools that contribute significantly to overall health. Their impact has been recognized by doctors such that in January 1945, the Colombia University College of Physicians and Surgeons established a Psychoanalytic and Psychosomatic clinic to study the unconscious mind and the relationship between the mind and the body. This was the first in the United States.

This book explores how embracing positive thinking and maintaining a positive mental attitude can be instrumental in fostering a healthy lifestyle and recovery from illness.

INTRODUCTION

Health is a state of complete physical, mental, and social well-being and not merely the absence of disease or infirmity.

-World Health Organization (WHO)

Man has always sought ways to remain healthy and to treat different diseases. This search has led to the discovery of diets, medicines, techniques, exercises, meditations, etc. As these discoveries evolve, the search beam also rested on the effect of our thoughts, imaginations, and attitudes on our bodies. Many studies have looked at the role of positive thoughts and optimism on mental and physical health.

An important discovery was made between happiness and health-positive emotions and their correlation with longevity among nuns. Nuns have many similarities in their lifestyles with a few differences in personality and outlook. This makes them an ideal population for this study which commenced in the 1930s. Cheerful nuns were found to live longer than their less cheerful counterparts. For example, 90% of the most cheerful quarter of nuns were alive at the age of 85, while only 34% of the least cheerful quarter lived to that age.

Also, 54% of the most cheerful fourth were alive at 94 as against 11% of the least cheerful. This was published in the Journal of Personality and Social Psychology in 2001.

Patients should be encouraged to cheer up as much as possible because optimism is a good strategy in healthcare. An American physician, Dr Patch Adams, makes patients happy through comedy. He and others have been praised for their efforts.

It is said that the average person has about 6,000 thoughts a day. Some of these thoughts are negative and cause negative emotions. Positive and negative thoughts and feelings affect our health.

Positive thinking is a powerful force that has been increasingly recognized for its profound impact on various aspects of human life, particularly on health. A positive mental attitude is the practice of identifying and focusing on the good in any situation. The link between a positive mindset and physical well-being has been explored in numerous studies. Their findings suggest that having a positive outlook can contribute significantly to overall health and longevity. Benefits of optimism and positive thinking include lower blood pressure, better pain tolerance, decreased incidence of heart attack, lower stress level, greater resistance to infections and longer life span.

Though happy thoughts are beneficial to health, the idea is not free of problems. Positive thinking should not be used as a substitute for effective treatment but rather as complementary. A middle-ground position should be adopted in healthcare. Ethics require that limits be set on the positive thinking trend that is becoming increasingly popular in healthcare because unrestricted optimism can lead to delusions.

Chapter 1

The power of suggestion

"It is better to be alone than in bad company."

-George Washington

A suggestion is an idea put forward for consideration. If your mind accepts the idea as true, your body responds accordingly. In an interesting study by Dalton, seventeen people who have asthma were divided into two groups. All participants were given the same pure rose scent to smell for 15 minutes. One group was told that it could make them breathe better, while the other was told that it could cause breathing difficulty. Guess the outcome? The first group liked the smell and had no reaction and no inflammation. The second group said that it made them feel sick and caused inflammation in their airways that lasted for 24 hours.

Family members and neighbours sometimes offer their opinions on how we can maintain health and treat illnesses. These information may be correct or simply misconceptions, despite the good intentions. The choice of place of healthcare can also be influenced by people around us. I have seen several patients who came to the hospital to receive treatment for one illness but refuse treatment for another health problem because they have been advised on where to get treatment for that kind of sickness. They may choose to seek care in spiritual/prayer houses or purchase medicine from a recommended patent medicine dealer who has successfully treated similar conditions.

One patient came on a follow-up visit. I noticed a one-sided weakness in gait as she made her way into the clinic. On inquiry, she said that she had suffered a stroke and is receiving care for it in a spiritual house. I suggested a referral to a neurologist but she declined because she had been advised that this kind of sickness needs spiritual therapy.

Many internal and external factors and their interplay influence the way we think about our health. These include childhood experiences and early conditioning. Messages received during formative years regarding health can significantly impact the thoughts we carry into later stages of life. The attitudes and behaviours of those around us, societal norms, and cultural influences contribute to the formation of beliefs about health and well-being. These external influences can either reinforce positive health behaviours or perpetuate detrimental thought patterns.

The internal dialogue or self-talk or **auto-suggestion** can either empower or hinder our well-being. Cultivating awareness of self-talk and intentionally adopting positive affirmations can redirect thought patterns toward a more health-conscious trajectory. Speak positive words to yourself, "I am healthy. I am strong. I feel great."

You can wish yourself sick and it will come to pass. I remember an incident that happened when I was very young. I wished that I would fall sick. I did that because I was upset about something and needed attention. I fell asleep in the afternoon only to wake up with a high fever. I have heard a similar story from another person who got sick just by wishing it to be so. Your body listens to your words and your thoughts.

Our ability to cope with challenges and adapt to stressors is intimately linked to the thoughts we generate. The generation of constructive thoughts is an effective coping mechanism that promotes health and resilience. On the other hand, negative thought patterns can contribute to the development or exacerbation of health issues.

Genetics also contribute to individual predispositions towards certain thought patterns. For example, individuals with a genetic predisposition to anxiety disorders may experience persistent anxious thoughts.

Recognizing the interconnected nature of these factors provides opportunities for targeted interventions, empowering individuals to cultivate positive thought patterns and in turn, enhance their overall well-being.

Chapter 2

Fear of Diseases – Nosophobia

"The real disease is fear. Throw the fear away and the disease will go."

-The Mother

From loudspeakers in markets and motor parks, I hear these kinds of marketing jingles - "Staph (staphylococcus) infection can be gotten from public toilets. It can cause bad dreams, persistent headaches, partial blindness, pre etc. To avoid these complications, buy our medicine." This information and others given by relatives, neighbours, friends, and well-meaning individuals can lead to fear of non-existent diseases. If a person is told repeatedly that he is sick, he will start experiencing symptoms of the disease.

Nosophobia is an intense irrational fear of developing a disease, usually a potentially life-threatening one, such as cancer, heart disease, HIV, etc. This worry tends to persist even after doctors have examined the individual and confirmed the absence of the disease. The person may experience physical symptoms like nausea, increased pulse rate, dizziness, sweating, rapid breathing, and sleeplessness.

Nosophobia is different from **hypochondria**, which is now known as **illness anxiety disorder**. While nosophobia involves the fear of developing a specific disease, illness anxiety disorder involves more general worries about illnesses. Someone with illness anxiety disorder may worry about minor symptoms, and see them as signs of something serious. Someone with nosophobia may worry about developing cancer or a brain tumor even when there are no symptoms.

People with nosophobia may make frequent trips to the doctor and request medical tests. Or they may develop a **fear of doctors (iatrophobia)** because they are afraid that they will diagnose a disease. They often feel that doctors do not take their symptoms and concerns seriously.

A related and fairly new phobia is **cyberchondria (or compuchondria).** This refers to people reading about a certain disease online (cyberspace) and then believing they have, or will get that disease. They search for medical information online and develop anxiety about their health following self-diagnosis. A survey found that more than 75% of participants in nine countries (Russia, China, India, Mexico, Brazil, United States, Italy, Australia, and Germany) use the internet for health-related information. Nearly 90% of adult Internet users in the United States reported searching for health information on the internet at least once. While access to online information about our health can be empowering and may help us to be aware of our health needs, googling symptoms can lead you to believe that you have a serious or even deadly health condition. Some patients go against medical advice or refuse to accept a professional diagnosis while quoting questionable web sources. This can be a frustrating obstacle to physicians trying to provide a professional standard of care.

Fears of illness and medical care are common in the general population. Illness/injury fears are often associated with lower income and education and in those with medical conditions. Interference with medical care also occurs among individuals with the strongest fears. These were findings of a study published in the Journal of Psychosomatic Medicine in 2000 titled, 'Illness Fears in the General Population'.

A symptom can mean different things. Headache can be caused by stress or hunger and will resolve after resting or having a meal. Headache can also be a symptom of other problems like excessive alcohol use, malaria, high blood pressure, meningitis, brain tumours, etc. If you have concerns about any symptoms, see your doctor. If you are not satisfied, seek a second opinion. Do not self-diagnose. Also, remain optimistic expecting the best outcome.

Chapter 3

Speaking Mind, Listening Body

"Your body hears everything your mind says."

-Naomi Judd

Thoughts have the power to shape our reality and influence our lives. Thoughts have an impact on our physical bodies and health. Various articles have shown that negative thoughts can lead to stress and anxiety with negative consequences on our bodies, while positive thoughts can lead to feelings of happiness and well-being with a positive impact on our bodies. It is important that we understand the power of our thoughts and be careful about what we think about and focus on.

The mind and body are intricately connected, and the state of one can influence the other. Scientific studies have demonstrated the impact of thoughts and emotions on physiological functions, immune system response, and overall health. It has been found that people with a positive mental attitude are more hopeful about life and would participate in healthful activities and follow doctors' recommendations.

A study done in California, USA found that having a positive mental attitude was linked to decreased mortality. People who had positive outlook were more likely to get regular physical exercise, avoid smoking, eat a healthier diet, and get more quality sleep. The results of the study also suggest that persons with negative attitudes have increased risk of death. These were the findings of a prospective cohort study where 13,674 participants were followed up over 35 years. The results were published in 2018 in the Journal of Aging Research.

Another study found that positive thinking can aid in the management of stress, and plays an important role in overall health and well-being. Higher optimism was found to be associated with a lower risk of death from many major causes which included cancer, heart disease, stroke, respiratory disease, and infections. This was a prospective cohort study carried out among 121,700 female registered nurses in the United States on the impact of optimism and cause-specific mortality. The result was published in the American Journal of Epidemiology in 2017.

The body often responds to commands and instructions from the mind. This relationship is central to the functioning of human physiology and psychology. For example, the brain sends signals through the nervous system to muscles, instructing them to contract or relax, enabling movement and coordination. The mind also controls involuntary bodily functions, such as heart rate, digestion, and respiratory rate. Emotions can significantly influence physical states. For example, stress can lead to increased heart rate and muscle tension, while relaxation can slow heart rate and reduce stress hormones.

Techniques like mindfulness, meditation, and yoga illustrate the power of the mind over the body. These practices can help manage pain, reduce stress, and improve overall well-being by focusing and directing mental attention. Mental states can manifest physically, such as in psychosomatic illnesses where psychological factors lead to physical symptoms.

Chapter 4

The Placebo and Nocebo Effects

"We tend to get what we expect."

-Norman Vincent Peale

The placebo effect is a phenomenon in which a person experiences real and noticeable improvements in symptoms or conditions after receiving a treatment that has no therapeutic effect. This response occurs because the individual believes the treatment to be effective. The placebo effect is often attributed to the psychological and physiological factors associated with the expectation of improvement. In many studies, patients who were given sugar pills (with no active ingredient) or saline injections but believed that they were receiving a potent pain medication, reported substantial reduction in pain.

Placebo effects are positive outcomes that occur following positive expectations, while **nocebo** effects are negative outcomes that are produced by negative expectations. Both effects occur because of what the patient believes to be true about the treatment, even though the treatment is inactive and harmless. Placebo effects can improve symptoms, while nocebo effects can worsen them. The placebo and nocebo effects are a prove that mindset affects health.

Fear can cause disease while expectation of healing can lead to quick recovery.

Numerous studies have shown that placebo effects are associated with the release of substances such as endogenous opioids, endocannabinoids, dopamine, oxytocin, and vasopressin. It is believed that expectation of relief causes this release. The effect of these substances is specific to the target system and the illness.

An article published in The New England Journal of Medicine in 2020 showed that the various ways patients experience symptoms and respond to treatments are partly due to placebo and nocebo effects. In many double-blind clinical trials of treatments for pain or psychiatric disorders, the responses to placebo are similar to the responses to active treatment, and up to 19% of adults and 26% of elderly persons taking placebos reported side effects. Also, as many as one-quarter of patients receiving placebo in clinical trials discontinue it because of side effects. This suggests that the nocebo effect may contribute to the discontinuation of or lack of adherence to active treatments.

A well-known and documented side effect of opioids is respiratory depression. In one study, placebo opioids were given to participants who had recently taken genuine opioids. The researchers found that the placebo drug elicited respiratory depression (nocebo effect), despite having no active ingredients.

Placebo surgeries (or sham surgeries) have been used to treat patients with surprising results. In one famous study, doctors performed knee surgeries (arthroscopic partial meniscectomy) for degenerative meniscal tear on some patients, while other patients received a small incision. The outcomes for the surgery were not better than those for the sham surgery. This was documented in The New England Journal of Medicine in 2013.

The placebo effect is strongly linked to the patient's belief in the treatment and the expectation that it will lead to improvement. The more a person believes in the effectiveness of a treatment, the more likely they are to experience positive outcomes.

The brain plays a significant role in the placebo effect. Positive thoughts and emotions can trigger the release of endorphins and other neurotransmitters, which may contribute to symptom relief. The placebo effect can lead to measurable physiological changes in the body. For example, a person may experience a reduction in pain perception, changes in heart rate, or improvements in other measurable health indicators.

The effectiveness of the placebo effect can be influenced by the context in which the treatment is administered. Factors such as the appearance of the treatment, the behaviour of healthcare providers, and the overall treatment environment can impact the strength of the placebo response. A systematic review of 12 published articles found that red, yellow, and orange colour on pills is associated with a stimulant effect, while blue and green are associated with a tranquilizing effect. This was published in the British Medical Journal in 1996.

While the placebo effect can lead to genuine improvements in symptoms, it raises ethical questions in medical practice. Providing a treatment that has no therapeutic value without the patient's knowledge is considered unethical. Informed consent and transparency are crucial in ethical medical care.

Hypnosis is another evidence of mind-body connection. The book, 'Psycho-Cybernetics' described an experiment where college students were told that they should imagine that one hand was immersed in ice water. The thermometer reading showed that the temperature dropped in that hand. Hypnotized individuals who are told that they are being touched by a very hot object, grimace with pain, their cardiovascular and lymphatic systems react and produce inflammation and sometimes blisters. The power of hypnosis is the power of belief. Dr Barbara explained that hypnotic subjects can do amazing things when they are convinced that the hypnotist's words are true statements. The subject behaves differently because he thinks and believes differently. It does not matter where the idea comes from. You may never have met a professional hypnotist. But if you have accepted an idea from people or advertisements and believe it to be true, it will have the same power over you as hypnotized subjects.

Hypnosis has been used to help in pain management, stress reduction, behavioural change like smoking cessation, and faster recovery from surgery and other medical procedures. It is important to note that while there is some evidence supporting the effectiveness of hypnosis in certain contexts, hypnosis is often used as a complementary therapy rather than a stand-alone treatment.

These effects and phenomena confirm the mind-connection that can and should be used in our favour.

Chapter 5

What to do when you are well

"I have chosen to be happy because it is good for my health."

-Voltaire

Thoughts, imaginations, beliefs, expectations, and attitudes all have a great impact on our health. "Thoughts are things", says Prentice Mulford. "Imagination creates reality", says Neville Goddard. "As a man thinks, so is he", (The Bible, Proverbs 23:7). Be careful about what you think about. You attract what you focus on. "Whatever is true, honourable, right, pure, lovely, admirable – if anything is excellent or praiseworthy – think on these things (Philippians 4:8, paraphrased). It is easier to think negative thoughts because we live in a negative world. But we can choose our thoughts.

Living positively involves cultivating a mindset and adopting behaviours that contribute to a more optimistic and fulfilling life. Take time each day to reflect on the things you are grateful for. This could be as simple as being thankful for supportive friends and family. Express gratitude for your body and its incredible capabilities. Appreciate your body functions that keep you alive and allow you to experience the world. Focus on what your body can do rather than dwelling on perceived shortcomings.

Challenge negative thoughts and replace them with positive ones. "Cast down imagination", (The Bible, 2 Corinthians 10:5). Focus on solutions rather than problems. Spend time with positive and supportive people. The energy and attitudes of those around you can have a significant impact on your outlook. Incorporate positive affirmations into your daily routine. Remind yourself of your strengths, resilience, and the potential for positive change. Say to yourself, "I am healthy and strong". Affirmations can help counter negative thoughts and build a more optimistic outlook.

Eating the right kinds of food. Choose foods that nourish your body and provide essential nutrients. Remember fresh fruits and vegetables. Be as close to nature as you can with your choice of diet. Choose fresh over processed food. Spend your money on the right kinds of food even if they are more expensive than processed food. Good health is your most important possession; more important than clothes. Stay hydrated, drink a lot of water. Find activities you enjoy, whether it's walking, dancing, or participating in other sports. Physical activity contributes not only to physical health but also to mental well-being.

Quality sleep is essential in maintaining overall health. Create a conducive sleep environment. Being active during the day helps you sleep well at night. "The sleep of a labouring man is sweet", (The Bible, Ecclesiastes 5:12). Even if you are elderly, get busy with something you love. There must be something you can do. If you sleep a lot during the day, you will stay awake at night.

Find joy in everyday activities. Find pleasure in simple moments, whether it is enjoying a glass of water or fruit juice, spending time with nature, or connecting with loved ones. Stay with people that make you happy. Keep as far as you possibly can from toxic relationships and high maintenance relationships. Do you know about 'High Maintenance Relationships'? I will share with you some of its attributes. You become anxious whenever you are about to meet that person or pick up his/her call. You worry about what happened in the last meeting, did you say or do things right? Every encounter seems to be an examination. The person is difficult to please. This type of relationship saps emotional energy from you and can also affect your health. You can find out more about High Maintenance Relationships.

Being joyful is a fundamental aspect of a healthy living. Remember the importance of social connections in promoting health. Foster positive relationships, share experiences, and seek support when needed. Strong social ties contribute to emotional well-being and a sense of belonging.

Incorporating health-promoting thoughts and activities into your daily life can contribute to a positive and balanced mindset, ultimately enhancing your overall well-being. Cultivating a healthy mindset is an ongoing process, and small, consistent steps can lead to significant positive changes over time.

As discussed earlier, positive mindset is closely linked to making healthier lifestyle choices. Individuals with an optimistic outlook are more likely to engage in activities that promote health, such as regular exercise, a balanced diet, and adequate sleep. Positive thinkers often view these choices as opportunities for self-care, leading to a more health-conscious and active lifestyle.

Chapter 6

What to do when you are sick

"Whether you think that you can or you think you can't, you're right."

-Henry Ford

Maintaining a positive attitude can play a crucial role in the recovery process. Studies indicate that patients with an optimistic outlook tend to recover more quickly from surgeries and illnesses. Positive thinking fosters resilience and a proactive approach to recovery influencing the body's healing mechanisms.

In the book, 'Anatomy of an Illness as Perceived by the Patient', Norman Cousins described his discovery of the therapeutic potential of laughter. He researched the biochemistry of human emotions which he believes is the key for fighting illness. He was diagnosed with ankylosing spondylitis, a crippling disease marked by severe inflammation in the spine often leading to a bedridden state; in addition to a severe connective tissue illness or collagen disease. He was told that he had a 1 in 500 chance of recovery. He took an active part in his own management, modifing his environment. He discovered that ten minutes of laughter while watching humorous movies gave him two hours of pain-free sleep without taking his analgesics. He made a remarkable recovery.

In the book, 'Psycho-Cybernetics', Dr. Maxwell Maltz, a renowned plastic surgeon, documented his observation of his patients who made a rapid recovery from surgery. Recognizable characteristics among all the rapid healers were optimism, cheerfulness, and positive thinking. They expected to get well and had some compelling reason to do so. They had something to look forward to in the future. Some people wanted to recover so that they could get back to work or attend an event.

Studies have shown that our sense organs work better when we are happy. We think better, see better, perform better, feel better, and are healthier. Dr William Bates proved that eyesight improves when the individual is thinking pleasant thoughts or visualizing pleasant scenes. Psychosomatic medicine has shown that our liver, stomach, heart, and all other organs function better when we are happy. Dr John A. Schindler said that unhappiness is the sole cause of all psychosomatic illnesses and that happiness is the only cure.

Be mindful of your self-talk. Repeat positive affirmations like "I am getting stronger every day". Replace negative or fearful thoughts with constructive and empowering ones. "Let the weak say, I am strong" (The Bible, Joel 3:10). Instead of dwelling on symptoms, focus on the healing process and your body's resilience.

Focus on the aspects of your health that are functioning well. Express gratitude for the parts of your body that are healthy and functioning optimally. Picture yourself in a state of complete well-being. Envision your body healing and cells rejuvenating. Visualization can have a powerful impact on your subconscious mind. Imagination creates reality. Put up a picture of yourself when you were well and full of life where you can see it. That is your desired destination.

Work with your healthcare provider to develop a recovery plan and follow it with a positive and proactive attitude. Adhere to your treatment plan. Healing takes time. Be patient with the process, and trust that your body is working towards recovery. Prioritize self-care practices that promote overall well-being. This includes adequate rest, a balanced diet, hydration, and activities that bring you joy and relaxation.

Be happy. “A cheerful heart is good medicine, but a crushed spirit dries up the bones” (The Bible, Proverbs 17: 22). Be hopeful, your attitude will affect the outcome.

Remember, while maintaining a positive mindset is beneficial, it is essential to combine it with appropriate medical care and guidance.

Chapter 7

How health workers can help

The good physician treats the disease, the great physician treats the patient who has the disease.

-William Osler

Health workers play a crucial role in supporting patients' mental well-being in addition to their physical health. Every health worker should offer some hope to the patient. And a smile. Although the doctor needs to tell the patients about the poor prognosis of ailments and obtain consent for treatment, some hope should be given. For example, a doctor can tell a patient, "This treatment has many potential side effects – you can become paralyzed, blind, or even die, and the success rate is 1%. You are the 1% that we have been waiting for." This positivity can improve treatment outcomes for health workers and hospitals.

On her first visit to the clinic, a patient asked me, "Doctor, will I die?" I replied, "If you were supposed to die, you would not have made it this far." I went ahead to tell her about other patients whose conditions were more severe than hers but had survived. She made a quick recovery. Often when she comes around for follow-up visits, she would request to say hello to me. She will simply say, "Doctor, do you remember me? I'm still alive!"

Health workers can help foster a positive mental attitude in their patients through effective communication. They should provide clear and accurate information about the patient's condition, treatment plan, and expected outcomes. Also, they should practice active listening to ensure patients feel heard and understood. Patients should be involved in their care by explaining treatment options and encouraging them to make informed decisions. Empowering patients can enhance their sense of control and positivity.

Acknowledge patients' emotions and concerns, showing that you care about their overall well-being. Create a welcoming and supportive healthcare environment. A positive and compassionate atmosphere can positively impact patients' mental states. If necessary, refer patients to mental health professionals or support groups. Mental health resources can complement medical treatment and offer additional support. Engage family members to the extent the patient approves. Respect and accommodate the patient's cultural and spiritual beliefs, to the extent that is possible. Health workers should recognize the importance of addressing the patient as a whole, including their beliefs and values.

We should celebrate treatment milestones and improvements. Positive reinforcement can motivate patients and contribute to a more optimistic outlook.

By integrating these strategies into their practice, health workers can contribute to a holistic approach to patient care that addresses both physical and mental well-being.

AFTERWORD

Think right, live right.

-Dr Paul R. Chipman

Our thoughts, imaginations and emotions play a vital role in our mental and physical health. We all experience negative thoughts and emotions at different times in our lives. Even the most resilient people experience fear, doubt, and anxiety. However, we can take charge of our minds and determine what to focus on. By embracing positivity, individuals can reduce stress, boost their immune systems, make healthier lifestyle choices, and effectively manage chronic conditions.

Positive thinking is being optimistic in any situation and expecting favourable outcomes. Social interactions play an important role in shaping our thoughts. It is important to be mindful of the power of suggestion and use it responsibly. Use auto-suggestion in your favour. Say what you would like to see. Your body hears your mind and your words. Fear can produce ill health, while the expectation of healing can lead to quick recovery.

As we navigate the complexities of life, cultivating a positive mindset is an essential component of a holistic approach to health. By harnessing the inherent strength of positive thinking, individuals can pave the way for a healthier, more fulfilling life.

In your imagination, see yourself well. Believe, heal and live. This is the winning mindset that produces success in all areas of life - career, finances, and everything else. Embrace it.

www.ingramcontent.com/pod-product-compliance
Lightning Source LLC
LaVergne TN
LVHW020526160826
845677LV00015B/3921

9798893836554